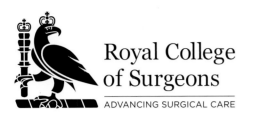

Surgical Skills for Students

Participant handbook

First edition (amended)

This handbook was written by Mr Rory McCloy, Mr Bill Thomas, Mr John Weston Underwood and Ms Louise Goldring

Published by The Royal College of Surgeons of England

Registered charity no: 212808

RCS Education

The Royal College of Surgeons of England

35–43 Lincoln's Inn Fields

London WC2A 3PE

Tel: 020 7869 6300

Fax: 020 7869 6320

Email: education@rcseng.ac.uk

Internet: www.rcseng.ac.uk

The Royal College of Surgeons of England would like to acknowledge the generous support of the following companies for their ongoing support of the College's course programme.

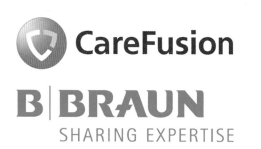
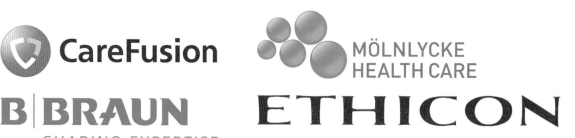

Contents

Introduction

This course is designed to teach you basic safe methods for performing simple surgical procedures and to allow you to perform and practise them on the bench using prepared animal tissue, simulations and various jigs. We aim to provide you with an enjoyable hands-on experience and the opportunity of practising vital and fundamental techniques in a skills lab environment. The aim of this course is to help you acquire good habits early in your career as it is so much harder to unlearn bad habits later in life. There is little essential preparation for the course apart from reading this handbook and watching the accompanying DVD.

Mr Rory McCloy FRCS

Basic Surgical Skills Development Tutor

The Royal College of Surgeons of England

Course objectives

- To learn safe operating techniques, gowning and gloving.
- To understand the characteristics and handling of surgical instruments.
- To learn the correct techniques for laying of safe surgical knots.
- To learn the correct techniques for commonly used sutures.
- To learn local anaesthetic techniques.
- To learn the basic principles of tissue dissection.

Part A

Principles of safe surgery (theatre safety)

- Always wear gloves of the correct size and choose appropriate gloves to suit the surgical procedure (see appendix).
- Never directly handle 'sharps'.
- Never handle a needle or scalpel blade with your fingers.
- When opening a needle packet, be careful to take the needle out of the specially designed packet using the needle holder and without touching the needle yourself.
- When changing the position of the needle in the needle holder, always use the forceps to change the orientation of the needle as demonstrated in the DVD. Once again, do not use your fingers.
- Always keep any needle in use within your direct sight at all times. When using a long suture length on your needle, utilise the middle finger of your right hand to control the long length, as shown in the DVD, and do not simply pull the needle out of view to tighten the suture material, as you can contaminate the needle or even injure your assistant.
- Always hand sharp instruments to assistants in a kidney dish or suitable container, to avoid injury. The safety of any assistant is the surgeon's responsibility.
- When changing the blade of a scalpel, be careful to handle the blade with forceps or haemostats. The blade is extremely sharp and should not be handled with your fingers.
- Always dispose of used needles or blades in the sharps container provided.
- Always dispose of excised tissue in the appropriate containers.
- Always keep the operative field tidy without extraneous instruments or equipment lying around.
- Operate with the table at the correct height – whether sitting or standing the height of the operative field should be approximately horizontal to your forearm **(Figure 1)**. Operating at any other height is likely to cause tiredness and stress.
- Throughout the course always wear aprons and gloves when handling tissues.
- Always dispose of gloves, theatre gowns and drapes in the appropriate manner.

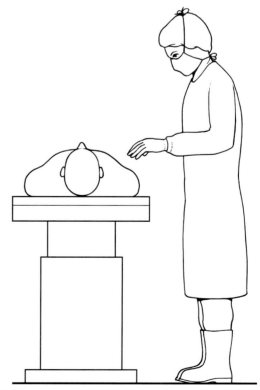

Figure 1

Gowning and gloving

The following procedure for putting on sterile theatre gowns and gloves is essential to the overall approach of operative sterile technique:

- Wash your hands thoroughly with appropriate antiseptic soaps (see appendix).
- Dry your hands from the hands down towards the elbows and then discard the towels.
- Pick up your gown and fold it so that the inside faces towards you.Put on the gown without touching the outside of the gown, keeping your hands inside the cuffs.
- Get an assistant to tie up the gown from the back.
- Open the glove packet.
- Use a closed gloving technique to put on your gloves **(Figures 2a to 2g)**.
- For a double-gloving technique, the first (inner) pair of gloves should be a half size larger than the correct size for your hands. The outer glove should be the correct size.
- Hand your assistant the tab of the posterior gown tie so that they handle only the tab end and not the tie itself. Turn around and then pull the tie out of the tab and tie it so that the posterior aspect of the gown is now closed.

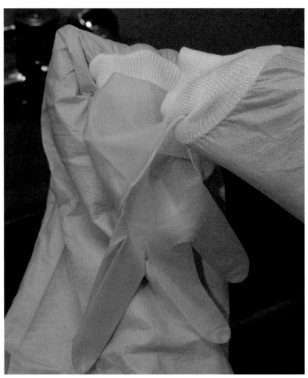

Figure 2a

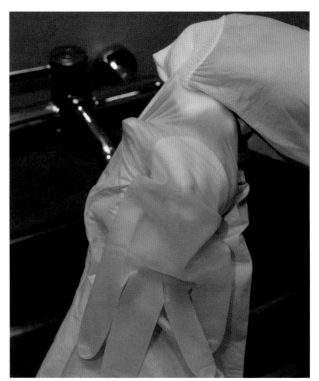

Figure 2b

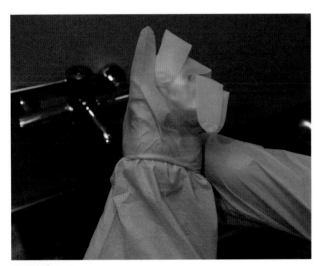

Figure 2c

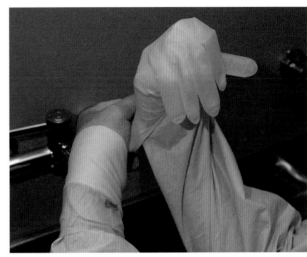

Figure 2f

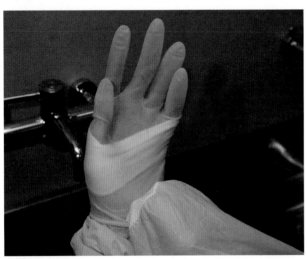

Figure 2d

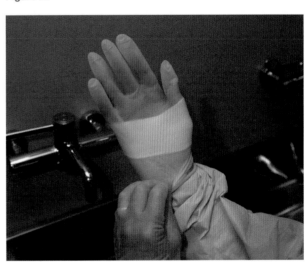

Figure 2g

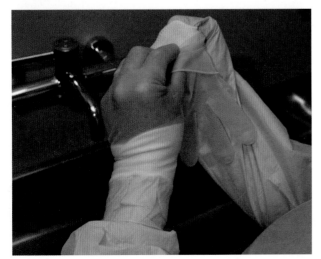

Figure 2e

Surgical safety and handling instruments

In order to achieve maximum potential from any surgical instrument it will need to be handled correctly and carefully. The basic principles of all instrument handling include:

- safety;
- economy of movement;
- relaxed handling;
- avoiding awkward movements.

We shall demonstrate the handling of scissors, haemostats, needle holders, forceps and scalpel. Take every opportunity to practise correct handling using the whole range of surgical instruments.

Scissors

Scissors are designed for use in the right hand. There are two basic types of scissors, one for soft tissues and one for firmer tissues such as sutures.

- Insert the thumb and ring finger into the rings (or bows) of the scissors so that just the distal phalanges are within the rings (Figure 3). Any further advancement of the fingers will lead to clumsy handling and difficulty in extricating the fingers at speed.
- Use the index finger to steady the scissors by placing it over the joint.
- When cutting tissues or sutures, especially at depth, it often helps to steady the scissors over the index finger of the other hand (Figure 4).
- Cut with the tips of the scissors for accuracy rather than using the crutch, which will run the risk of damaging tissues beyond the item being divided and will also diminish accuracy.

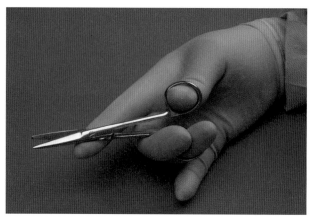

Figure 3

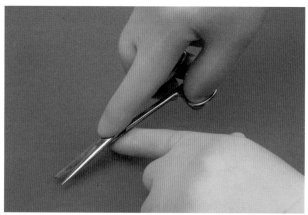

Figure 4

Haemostats (artery forceps)

Haemostats are designed primarily for use in the right hand. Haemostats may be curved or straight.

- Hold haemostats in a similar manner to scissors.
- Place on vessels using the tips of the jaws (the grip lessens towards the joint of the instrument).
- Secure position using the ratchet lock.
- Learn to release the haemostat using either hand. For the right hand, hold the forceps as normal, then gently further compress the handles and separate them in a plane at right angles to the plane of action of the joint. Control the forceps during this manoeuvre to prevent them from springing open in an uncontrolled manner. For the left hand, hold the forceps with the thumb and index finger grasping the distal ring and the ring finger resting on the under surface of the near ring (Figure 5). Gently

compress the handles and separate them again at right angles to the plane of action, taking care to control the forceps as you do so.

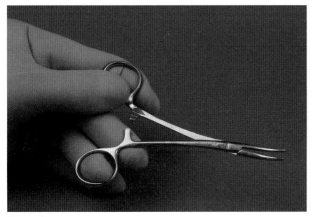

Figure 5

Needle holder

Needle holders are designed primarily for use in the right hand.

- A needle holder differs from a haemostat by way of the diamond-shaped milling of the 'teeth' which allows the shaft of a needle to be held securely at any angle **(Figure 6)**. The jaws may be lined with a harder metal than the steel of a needle shaft to prevent wear and damage to the instrument.

- Grasp the needle holders in a manner similar to scissors.

- Hold the needle in the tip of the jaws about two thirds of the way along its circumference **(Figure 7)**, never at its very delicate point and never too near the swaged eye.

- Select the needle holder carefully. For delicate fine suturing use a fine short-handled needle holder and an appropriate needle. Suturing at depth requires a long-handled needle holder.

- Most needle holders incorporate a ratchet lock but some (eg Gilles) do not. Practise using different forms of needle holder to decide which is most applicable for your use.

- There are a wide variety of needle and suture materials available and their use will depend on the tissues being sutured and the nature of the anastomosis.

- Practise the correct handling of each of the instruments (scissors, haemostats and needle holders) as demonstrated.

- Use the right hand first and then find out the limitations of using these instruments in the left hand.

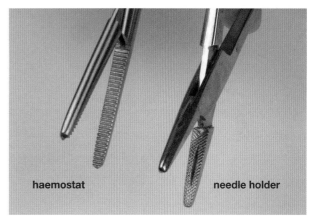

haemostat   needle holder

Figure 6

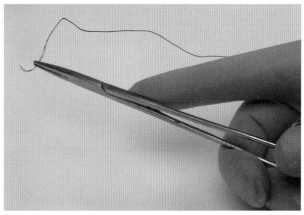

Figure 7

Dissecting forceps

- Hold gently between thumb and fingers, with the middle finger playing the pivotal role **(Figure 8)**.
- Two main types of forceps are available: toothed for tougher tissue such as fascia or skin, and nontoothed (atraumatic) for delicate tissues such as bowel and vessels.
- Toothed forceps should not be used on tubular tissues as they can cause holes and potentially a leak.
- A third type of forceps are called Debakey **(Figure 9)** and have special longitudinal grooves and ridges with milling. which can grip tissues and needles.
- Never crush tissues with the forceps but use them to hold or manipulate tissues with great care and gentleness.

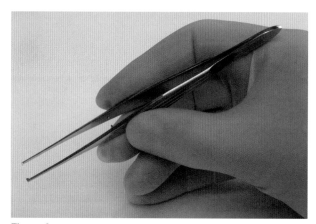

Figure 8

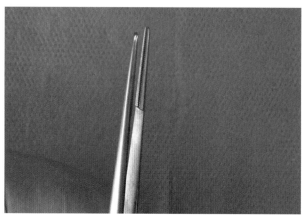

Figure 9

Scalpel

- Handle with great care as the blades are very sharp. Never handle the blade directly. When attaching the blade to the handle the haemostat must not cross the cutting edge of the blade or else it will blunt or burr the blade. The angle at the base of the blade must be matched with the angled slot on the handle so that the blade can slide down the groove in the handle and lock in place **(Figure 10)**. When removing the blade from the handle never point the tip down to the surgical drapes, as the patient beneath may be injured. The same applies to pointing the tip upwards or sideways because it may injure an assistant or yourself. Only remove the blade down onto the instrument trolley or into a suitable container.
- Practise attaching and detaching the blade using a haemostat.
- For making a routine skin incision hold the scalpel in the palm of the hand, with your index finger guiding the blade. Keep the scalpel handle horizontal and the blade at right angles to the tissues to prevent shearing of the tissue edges. Then draw the whole length of the sharp blade, not just the point, over the tissues **(Figure 11)**.
- For finer work the scalpel may be held like a pen, often steadying the hand by using the little finger as a fulcrum **(Figure 12)**.
- Always pass the scalpel in a kidney dish. Never pass the scalpel point first across the table.

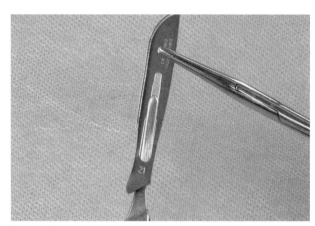

Figure 10

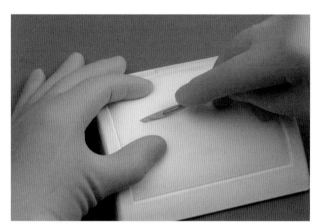

Figure 11

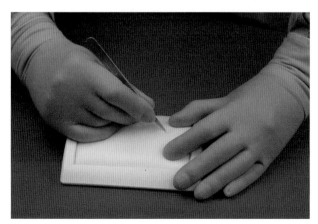

Figure 12

Knot tying

Knot tying is one of the most fundamental techniques in surgery and is often performed very badly. Take time to perfect your knot-tying technique as this will stand you in good stead for the rest of your career. Practise regularly with spare lengths of surgical thread.

General principles of knot tying include:
- The knot must be firm and unable to slip.
- The knot must be as small as possible to minimise foreign material.
- During tying do not 'saw' the material as this will weaken the thread.
- Do not damage the thread by grasping it with artery forceps or needle holders, except at the free end when using an instrument tie.
- Avoid excess tension during tying as this could damage the structure being ligated or even cause breakage of the thread.
- Avoid tearing the tissue that is being ligated by controlling tension at 'bedding down' of the knot, very carefully using the index finger or thumb as appropriate.

You will be taught and asked to demonstrate the following:
- the one-handed reef knot;
- an instrument-tied reef knot;
- the surgeon's knot;
- tying at depth.

When practising, tie your knots vertically over 'the wound', not down towards your lap. Standing up to tie knots is more representative of most surgical practices.

One-handed reef knot

A one-handed reef knot, properly thrown and laid, is the cornerstone of surgery. You will perform it with your left hand because your right hand may be holding the needle holder and also because it is easier to transfer your skills to your right hand later. Both throws are tied with the hands over the wound and are held horizontally. The one-handed reef knot consists of two throws, the coming down and the going up throw, performed alternately.

Coming down throw

If the short end of the thread leads away from you, perform the coming down throw first.
- Begin by bending the left elbow with the palm down and hand pointing towards you.
- Pick up the short end between the thumb and ring finger **(Figure 13a)**.
- Now turn the hand palm upwards so that the thread passes downwards over your straightened index and middle fingers **(Figure 13b)**.
- Next separate your thumb and ring finger from the middle and index fingers.
- With your right hand hold the long end of the thread (which may have a needle attached to it) and pass it up over the left middle and index fingers, thus creating a loop in the thread **(Figure 13c)**.
- Flex the left middle finger under the short end **(Figure 13d)** and then straighten the finger so that the short end is on the back of the middle finger and grip the short end between the middle and index fingers **(Figure 13e)**.
- The thread can now be released by the left ring finger and thumb and drawn through the loop with the middle and index fingers **(Figure 13f)**.
- Carefully lay the knot square.
- The hands have crossed and the ends are held 180° apart **(Figure 13g)**.
- The knot is then snugged down but do not let go of the suture with either hand.
- Now change the direction of the short end in the left hand by reversing it in the fingers **(Figure 13h)** and move the left hand behind the thread so that it lies over the knot rather than in your lap **(Figure 13i)**.

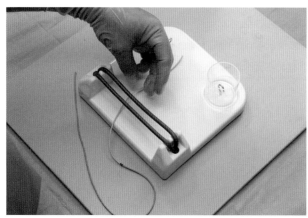

Figure 13a

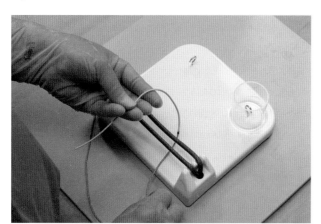

Figure 13b

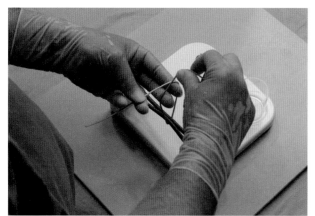

Figure 13c

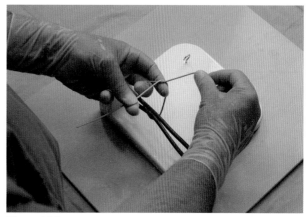

Figure 13d

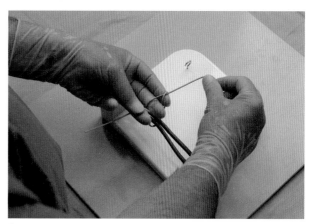

Figure 13e

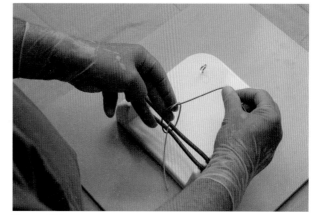

Figure 13f

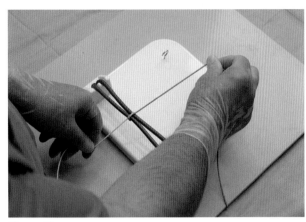

Figure 13g

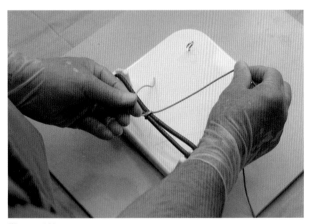

Figure 13h

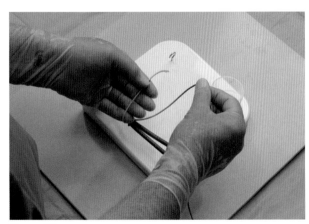

Figure 13i

Going up throw

When you did the coming down throw, you finished with the thread held between your left thumb and index finger with the thread passing from them over the hand.

- Now turn the hand palm upwards so that the short end is passing upwards over your fingers towards the thumb and index finger, which are now separated from the remaining fingers **(Figure 13j)**.

- With the right hand, which is still holding the long end of the thread away from you, pass it downwards over the left middle finger, creating the loop **(Figure 13k)**.

- The right hand comes right down towards you and stays there.

- By flexing the left middle finger under the short end, you can catch the end of the short thread on the back of the finger **(Figure 13l)** and straighten it so that the thread can be gripped between the middle and ring fingers **(Figure 13m)**.

- Release with the thumb and draw the short end through the loop **(Figure 13n)**.

- Lay it down carefully so that the going up short end continues to go on up and the hands have crossed in opposite directions **(Figure 13o)**.

- Finally snug it down. You can now see the typical figure of eight of a properly thrown reef knot **(Figure 13p)**.

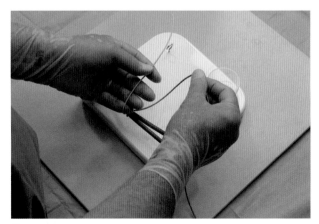

Figure 13j

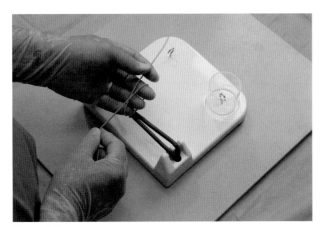

Figure 13k

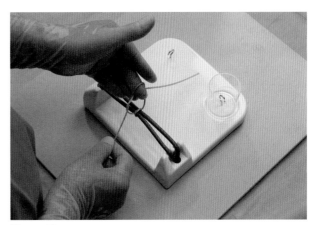

Figure 13n

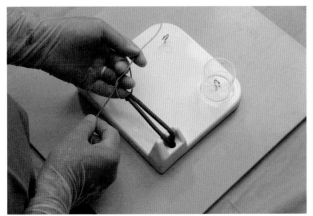

Figure 13l

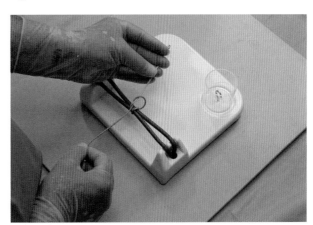

Figure 13o

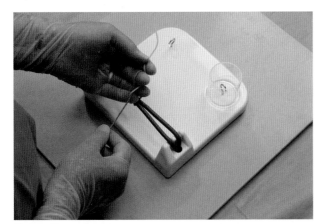

Figure 13m

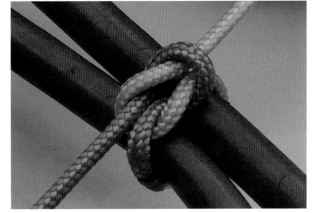

Figure 13p

You will notice that it is important that your hands move towards and away from you alternately with each throw. With a braided suture, which has a rough surface that will grip in the knot, it is usually sufficient to perform three alternating throws but with a smooth monofilament suture, which can slip easily and come undone, six throws are required.

Instrument tie

- Start by placing the instrument over the thread with the short end farthest away from you **(Figure 14a)**.
- Loop the long end of the thread up and over and around the instrument **(Figure 14b)**.
- Grasp the short end of the thread within the jaws of the instrument **(Figure 14c)**.
- Complete the first throw by pulling the short end down towards you and crossing your hands **(Figure 14d)**.
- Now place the instrument over the thread again with the short end nearest to you **(Figure 14e)** and form a loop around the instrument by bringing the long end down and over and around the instrument **(Figure 14f)**.
- With the instrument through the loop grasp the short end again within the jaws of the instrument **(Figure 14g)**.
- Pull through and cross the hands to complete the classical reef knot **(Figure 14h)**.

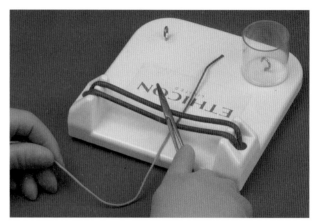

Figure 14a

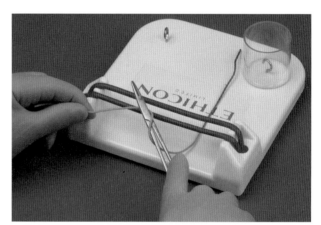

Figure 14b

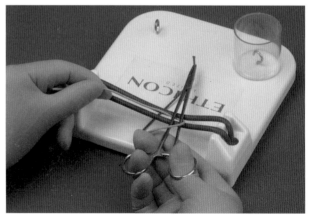

Figure 14c

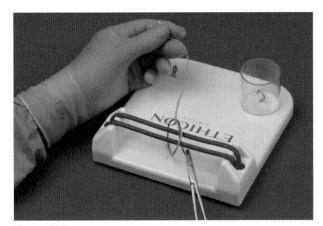

Figure 14d

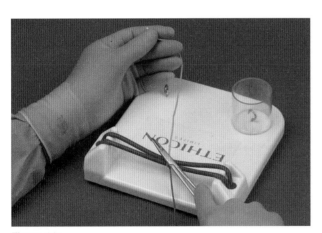

Figure 14e

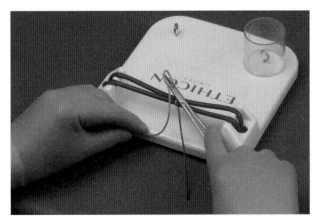

Figure 14f

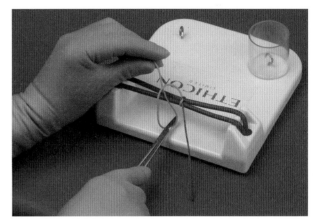

Figure 14g

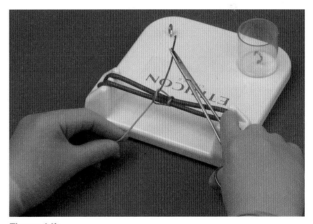

Figure 14h

Surgeon's knot

Sometimes we want a knot that is secure and will not slip between throws. To increase the friction in the first throw we can tie a double throw first and snug that down, and then return by a single throw. Although we do not have a very pretty looking knot, we have a very secure surgeon's knot.

- Begin in the same way as you did for the coming down throw of a single handed knot with your left hand, but hold the long end that is in your right hand as though it were about to perform a going up throw (**Figure 15a**).

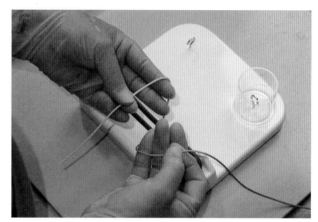

Figure 15a

- Separate the middle and ring fingers of the left hand.
- Form a loop by moving the right hand away from you over the middle and index fingers of the left hand so that your left index and middle fingers pass through the loop as usual (**Figure 15b**).
- Then pass the middle ring and little fingers of the right hand through the same loop (**Figure 15c**) with the palm upwards above the left index finger (**Figure 15d**).
- Bend both middle fingers under their respective ends of the thread and then straighten them so that the thread is on the back of each middle finger (**Figure 15e**).

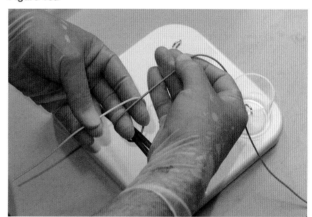

Figure 15b

- Using the index and middle fingers of the left hand, take the short end through the loop towards the left (**Figure 15f**) and at the same time take the long end through the loop towards the right using the middle and ring fingers of the right hand.
- Ensure the throw lies correctly by moving the left short end down towards you and the right long end away from you so that the hands cross (**Figure 15g**).
- Tighten appropriately (**Figure 15h**).
- Now perform a standard second single throw by doing a going up throw with the left hand (**Figures 15i to 15k**).

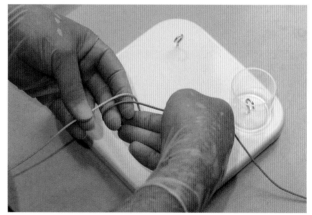

Figure 15c

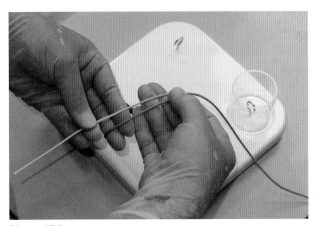

Figure 15d

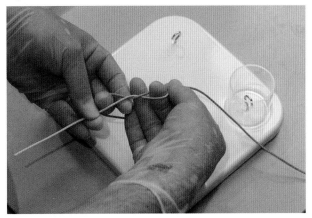

Figure 15e

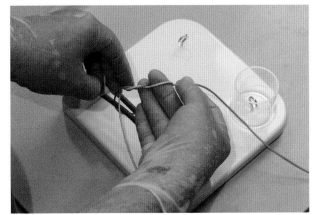

Figure 15f

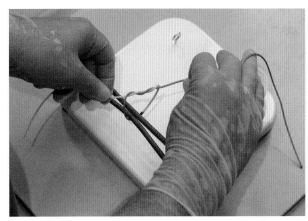

Figure 15g

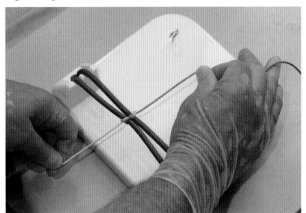

Figure 15h

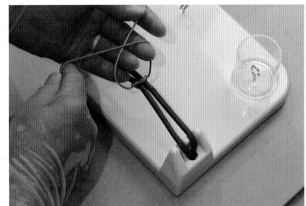

Figure 15i

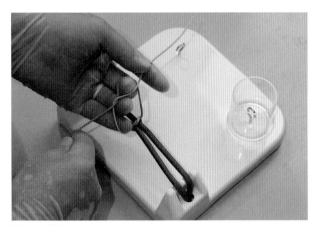

Figure 15j

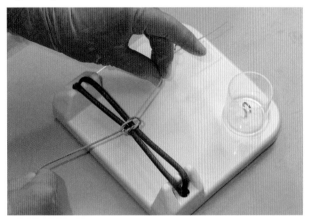

Figure 15k

Step-by-step practice:

- Hold the upper end as for a coming down throw with your left hand and lower end as for a going up throw with your right hand.
- Form a loop over the left middle finger.
- Pass the free fingers of the right hand through the loop.
- You are now set up to make the double throw.
- Bend both middle fingers to catch the thread ends.
- Draw both ends through and lay the knot square.

This technique of tying a surgeon's knot cannot be used if you have an instrument in the right hand. Be careful if there is a needle on the long end as it passes through the loop.

Instrument-tied surgeon's knot

To tie a surgeon's knot with an instrument, start as for a simple reef knot, but after passing the thread over and under the instrument, pass it over and under again forming a double loop (**Figure 16a**), before picking up the short end and passing it through the double loop (**Figure 16b**).

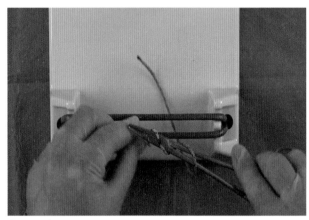

Figure 16a

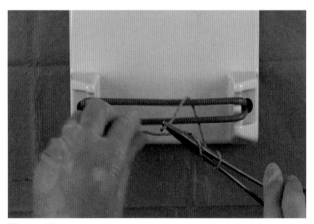

Figure 16b

Suturing techniques 1

When opening a suture package, tear it open as shown and remove the needle from the packet with the needle holder. Never use your fingers. Never pick up needles with your hands; it is important not to handle needles directly. When picking up needles use the needle holder and then if you wish to alter the position of the needle in the needle holder do not use your fingers but instead use the forceps to hold the needle and reposition it. Always pick up the needle with the forceps, then pick up the needle holder in a similar manner to the scissors and the haemostat. Place the needle holder about two-thirds of the way around the circumference of the needle. Grip the needle within 2 mm of the tips of the needle holders jaws.

Insertion of sutures requires a smooth supination of the forearm but occasionally a backhand suture is required, in which case the needle position can be changed in the needle holder, enabling you to insert a backhand suture. One arm pronates while the other arm supinates and therefore the needle can be changed from the forehand to the backhand very simply and efficiently. When you have finished with the needle do not lay it down on the patient or on the table but pick it up and, whenever possible, dispose of it by cutting off the thread and placing it in the sharps bin provided.

Basic principles

- Attempt to remove all elements of tension from any anastomosis.
- Insert the needle at right angles to the tissue and gently advance through the tissue, avoiding shearing forces.
- As a rough rule of thumb, the distance from the edge of the wound should correspond to the thickness of the tissue and successive sutures should be placed at twice this distance apart, ie at approximately double the depth of the tissue sutured **(Figure 17)**.

- All sutures should be placed at right angles to the line of the wound at the same distance from the wound edge and the same distance apart to ensure equal tension down the wound length. The only situation where this should not apply is when suturing fascia or aponeuroses, when the sutures should be placed at varying distances from the wound edge to prevent the fibres parting **(Figures 18a and 18b)**.

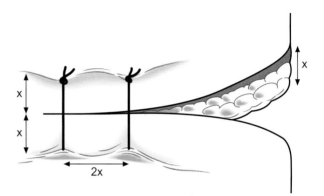

Figure 17

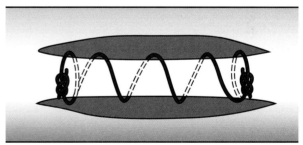

Figure 18a

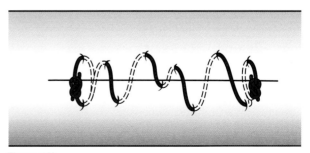

Figure 18b

- For closing long wounds with interrupted sutures, it is advisable to place the first stitch in the middle of the wound and subsequent stitches half way along that length and so on.
- No suture should be tied under too much tension otherwise subsequent oedema of the wound may cause the sutures to cut out or to cause ischaemia of the wound edge and delayed healing.
- In most cases it is advisable to only go through one edge of the tissues at a time but, if the edges lie in very close proximity and accuracy can be ensured, it is permissible to go through both edges at the same time.
- The edges of elliptical wounds, following lesion excision, may be undermined to help closure. However, the length of the wound will need to be approximately three times the width of the wound if closure is to be safe and not under too much tension. Skin hooks may be useful to display the wound.

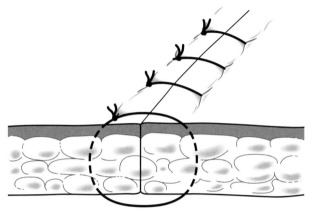

Figure 19

Types of suturing

You will be taught and asked to demonstrate the following types of suturing:

- interrupted sutures
- continuous sutures
- vertical mattress sutures
- subcuticular sutures

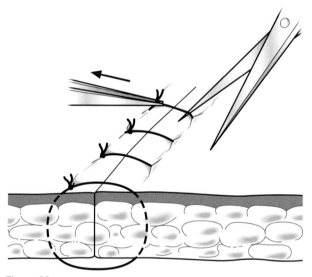

Figure 20a

Interrupted sutures (Figure 19)

- Place these carefully at right angles to the wound edges.
- Tie a careful reef knot and lay it to one side of the wound.
- Cut suture ends about 0.5 cm long to allow enough length for grasping when removing.
- When removing sutures, cut flush with the tissue surface so that the exposed length of the suture (which may be infected) does not have to pass through the tissues (**Figures 20a and 20b**).

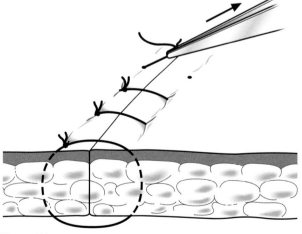

Figure 20b

Continuous sutures (Figure 21)

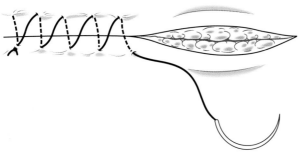

Figure 21

- Place a single suture and ligate but only cut the short end of the suture.
- Continue to place sutures along the length of the wound. Tension is kept equal by means of an assistant 'following' you, holding the suture at the same tension that it is handed to them at.
- Take care not to 'purse-string' the wound by using too much tension.
- Take care not to produce too much tension by using suture that is too short.
- Secure the suture at the end of the wound by a further reef knot

Vertical mattress sutures (Figure 22)

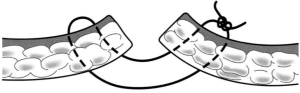

Figure 22

- They may be useful for ensuring eversion of a wound edge (Figure 22).

Part B

Reprise of knot tying

Common faults

- A correctly laid reef knot requires alternating throws of coming down and going up throws, crossing the hands with each throw.
- However, if we do a coming down throw and our right hand fails to move up and away, the left hand fails to continue coming down and we will not have the correct throw for a reef knot.
- If we do a coming down throw and cross our hands correctly but follow with another coming down throw, we will not have a reef knot even though we crossed our hands.
- If a coming down throw is being correctly formed and laid, and a going up throw is correctly formed but the right hand fails to move down so the left hand fails to continue going up, again, we do not have a reef knot. Always remember to cross your hands.
- A correctly laid reef knot requires alternating throws of coming down and going up throws, crossing the hands with each throw.
- One other common fault is for the surgeon to hold up one end of the suture with too much tension. While alternating throws are formed, they are not correctly laid because the right hand is not crossing. The vertical thread passes straight through the knot, which can slip, and the vertical thread can be pulled straight back through the knot.

Single handed surgeon's knot

- Start off in the same way as you would for a simple coming down throw.
- Pick up the short end and have it coming down over your fingers (Figure 23a).

- Hold it over the wound and separate the ring finger from the other two.
- Simply hold the right hand thread and pass it up over your hands (Figure 23b), then pass it up over your hands again to make a second loop (Figure 23c).
- Now you bend the middle finger, grip it between the index and middle (Figure 23d), and pull the thread through both loops at once and as you tie it down there are the two loops on the surgeon's knot.
- Finish off, as before, by a going up throw to lock it and then a further coming down throw so you've thrown a reef knot on top of a surgeon's knot.

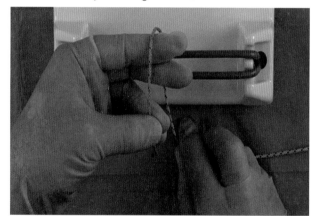

Figure 23a

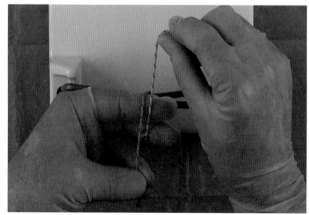

Figure 23b

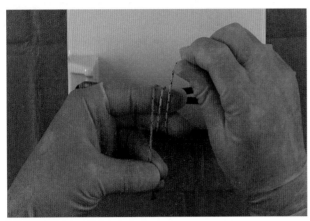

Figure 23c

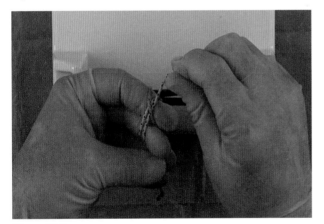

Figure 23d

Tying at depth

When tying a suture at depth, the alternating throws are identical to those in a one-handed reef knot but the crossing of the hands now has to be done in a vertical plane.

- With a haemostat pass the suture around the hook **(Figure 24a)**.
- If performing the coming down throw first **(Figure 24b)**, make the throw above the pot with your left hand and lead it down into the pot with your left index finger **(Figure 24c)**, taking the short end deeper than the hook **(Figure 24d)**, on the side nearest to you.
- Snug the throw by applying tension with the right hand vertically upwards and the left index finger vertically downwards.
- Now do the going up throw outside the pot **(Figure 24e)** and lead the throw down into the pot with your right index

finger **(Figure 24f)** taking the suture beyond the hook again **(Figure 24g)** on the side nearest to you. Complete the knot with another coming down throw.

- Snug down, again maintaining equal tension 180° apart in the vertical plane. A third throw may be added.
- When tying at depth, it is very important that the first throw does not come loose on the tissue whilst the second throw is being made and laid. For this reason it is common practice that the majority of ligatures at depth use a surgeon's knot on the first throw. This is best achieved by the single-handed surgeon's knot technique (described above in **Figures 23a to 23d**).

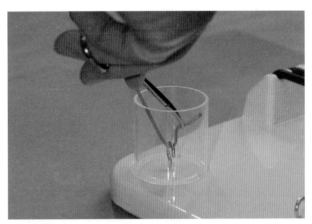

Figure 24a

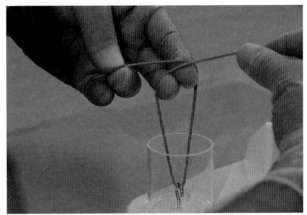

Figure 24b

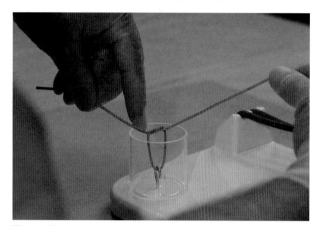

Figure 24c

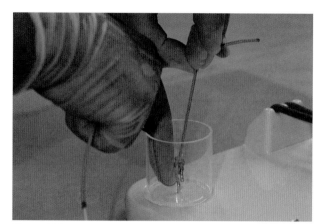

Figure 24f

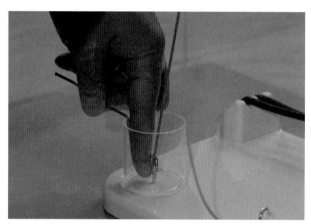

Figure 24d

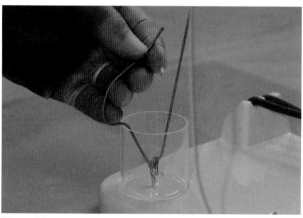

Figure 24g

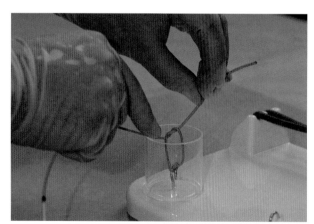

Figure 24e

Skin lesions

Local anaesthetic technique

Safe doses of lignocaine

The maximum safe dose of lignocaine is 3 mg/kg (6 mg/kg with adrenaline). The standard ampoule of 1% lignocaine contains 10 mg/ml. Therefore, the usual safe total volume of 1% lignocaine to be infiltrated in a 70 kg patient is 21 ml.

- Before excising a skin lesion you can practise the administration of local anaesthetic to the planned area of excision (best marked out with a suitable pen).
- There are two techniques. The first 'static' technique involves inserting the needle at the site of instillation and aspirating to make sure the tip is not in a blood vessel – no 'flash-back' of blood. It is then safe to inject the local anaesthetic as inadequate intravenous injection could lead to cardiac dysrhythmias **(Figure 25)**.
- The second technique involves continuous movement of the needle through the tissues while injecting the local anaesthetic. Any passage through a blood vessel would be transient and momentary and intravenous injection of any volume would not occur.
- It is kinder to start with a fine-bore needle until the initial area has been anaesthetised and then change to a longer, large-bore needle for infiltration of the planned surgical field.
- Check the planned area of incision has been successfully anaesthetised by gently touching with the tip of the scalpel blade and asking the patient if there is any sensation, before making a full incision.

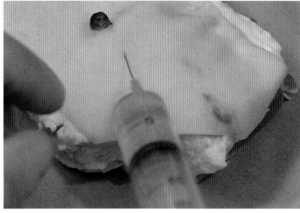

Figure 25

Elliptical excision

- Identify the skin lesion for excision and, assuming it to be benign, leave a 1-mm margin either side. Estimate the planned width. Then calculate the length of the elliptical excision as three times the width. This is the minimum width to length ratio for a cosmetic closure without undue tension **(Figure 26)**.
- If the area allows, then a 1:4 width to length ratio is even better.
- The use of a suitable skin marker may help plan the area and ensure the correct field for excision is infiltrated with local anaesthetic.
- After local anaesthesia has been achieved, excise an ellipse of skin, complete with lesion, and a portion of subcutaneous tissue shaped like the hull of a boat – this helps the skin to be closed without tension and avoids any risk of leaving part of the lesion deep to the skin if it had penetrated the dermis **(Figure 27)**.
- Close the skin with interrupted vertical mattress sutures starting at alternate ends and working towards the centre.

width × 1

length = 3 × width —— 1 mm margin

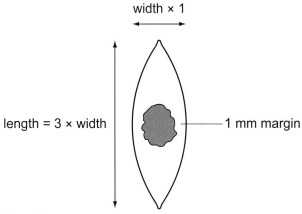

Figure 26

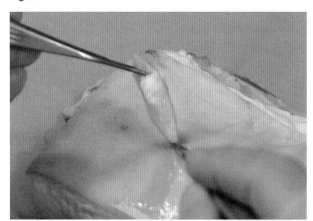

Figure 27

Suturing techniques 2

Subcuticular sutures (Figure 28)

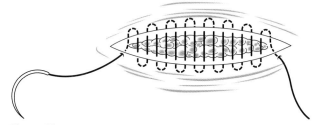

Figure 28

- Subcuticular sutures are a snake-like continuous suture in the horizontal plane of the skin as opposed to a vertical spiral plane of the previous sutures.
- This technique may be used with absorbable or non-absorbable sutures.
- Small bites are taken of the subcuticular tissues, the dermis, on alternate sides of the wound, which are then pulled carefully together.

Excision of sebaceous cyst

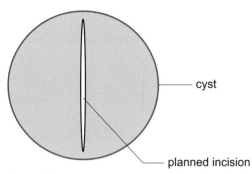

Figure 29a

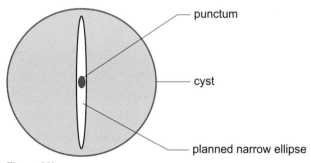

Figure 29b

- Identify the 'sebaceous cyst' in your model **(Figure 29a)**.
- Plan a linear incision over the 'roof' of the cyst which is no longer than the diameter of the cyst. If a 'punctum' is visible, induce this in your incision by taking a very narrow ellipse of skin **(Figure 29b)**.
- Work carefully through the subcutaneous tissues, using a combination of blunt and sharp dissection techniques, until the 'capsule' of the cyst is reached. Then carefully work round all sides staying close to the capsule – avoid puncturing the cyst!
- Close the skin with either interrupted simple sutures or a subcuticular suture.

Appendix

Scrubbing up

The choice of surgical scrub and gloves is critically important to a surgeon. This point is often not fully realised or appreciated.

Surgical handwashing

Surgical handwashing using approved scrub solutions is a technique that involves an initial washing of the hands and forearms, which removes transient micro-organisms and reduces the count of resident flora, and a second wash that further reduces the level of resident colonising flora.

Traditionally a sterile brush was used for the first application of the day but continual use is inadvisable as damage to the skin may occur. New alcohol-based formulations have been found to be suitable for use for surgical hand scrub and for brushless application.

Alcohol antiseptics are as effective and have as wide a spectrum of antimicrobial activity as the more conventional methods using antiseptic detergent solutions and are no more damaging to the skin. Therefore, scrub solutions should be chosen that:

- have substantial initial reduction of transient and resident flora;
- are effective against a wide spectrum of micro-organisms;
- have a persistent effect and will continue to work after application (in case of glove puncture);
- are not damaging to the skin.

Handwashing technique (4 minutes)

- Adjust the water temperature, then the flow to avoid splashing.
- During washing, keep your arms in front of you with the hands higher than the elbows so the water runs down away from the hands and off at the elbows (**Figure 30a**).
- Dispense the antimicrobial solution with the elbow (**Figure 30b**).
- Rub the hands palm to palm (**Figure 30c**).
- Rub your left palm over right dorsum of hand and repeat with right palm over left dorsum (**Figure 30d**).
- Rub palm to palm with fingers interlaced (**Figure 30e**).
- Rub backs of fingers with the opposing palms with the fingers interlocked (**Figure 30f**).
- Grasp the thumb with the opposing hand and rub by rotating the hand (**Figure 30g**). Repeat with the other thumb and hand.
- Rub the palm of each hand with the clasped fingers of the opposing hand (**Figure 30h**).
- Rub the left wrist and arm to within a few centimetres of the elbow using the right hand (**Figure 30i**). Repeat for the other arm.
- If the scrub is the first of the session, brush under the nails but avoid the skin (**Figure 30j**).
- Wash the forearms again but stop one third of the way from the elbow (**Figure 30k**).
- Rinse the hands and arms thoroughly, keeping the hands up so the water runs down to the elbows (**Figure 30l**).
- At arm's length use the first towel to dry one hand and arm. Pat, not rub, the skin dry working towards the elbow (**Figure 30m**).
- Drop the towel when you reach the elbow. Repeat using the second towel for the other arm (**Figure 30n**).

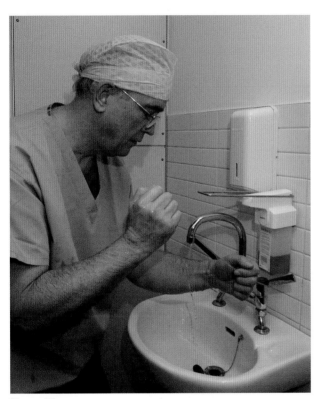

Figure 30a

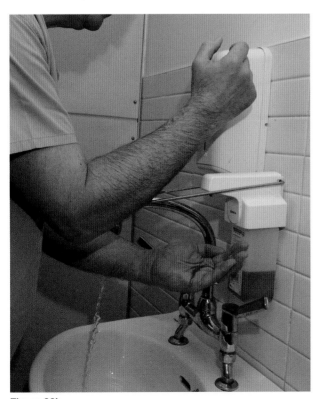

Figure 30b

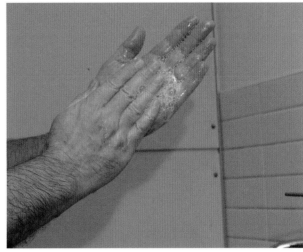

Figure 30c

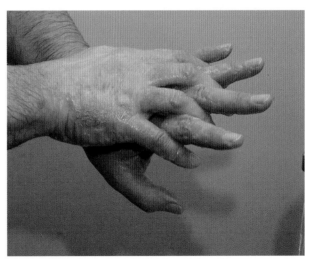

Figure 30d

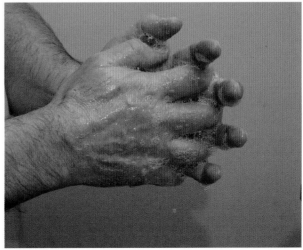

Figure 30e

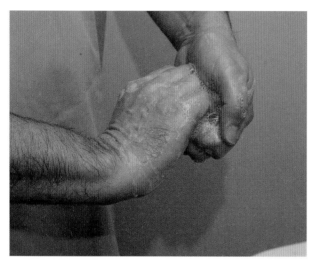

Figure 30f

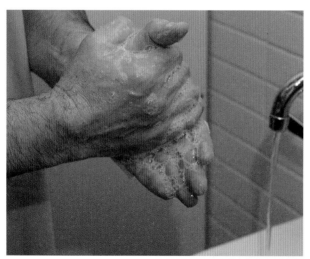

Figure 30g

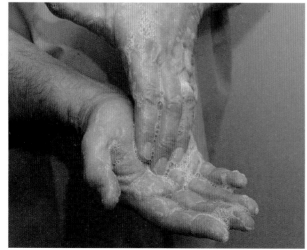

Figure 30h

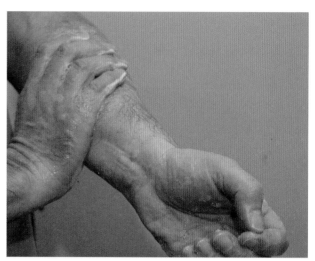

Figure 30i

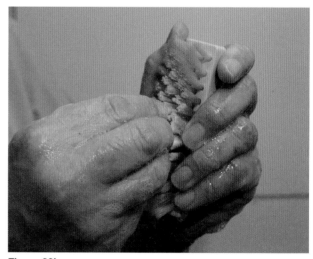

Figure 30j

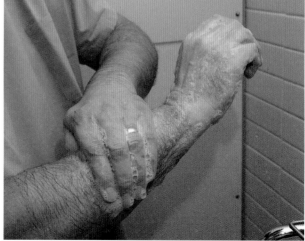

Figure 30k

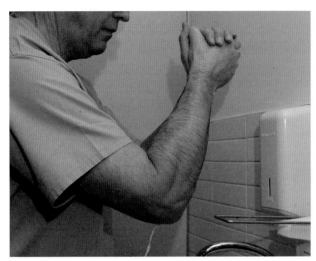

Figure 30l

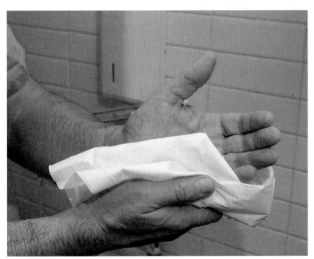

Figure 30m

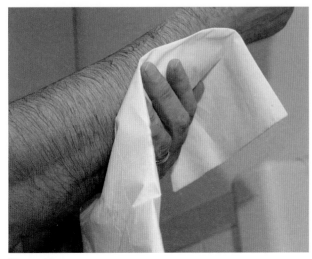

Figure 30n

Choice of gloves

Given the length and complexity of many operations it is obvious that gloves must fit securely and offer optimum sensitivity and durability without causing hand fatigue. They should not lose their shape or integrity during use.

Less well understood is the need for the gloves to be of high quality, low in extractable latex proteins and powder-free. It is well documented that adhesions and other postoperative complications including delayed wound healing can be attributed to glove powder which transfers latex proteins from the surface of the glove.

The surface of the glove must also be low in residual accelerators used in the manufacturing process because these can cause localised skin conditions, sometimes occurring up to 48 hours after contact. With increased usage of latex gloves the incidence of latex allergy in the US has risen to between 28% and 67% in some high-risk healthcare workers and is estimated to affect 6% of the general population. Latex allergy often takes time to develop; there can be months or even years of exposure before any reaction occurs. Although latex is still recognised as the best barrier, latex-free alternatives should be considered when sensitisation occurs to the proteins in natural rubber latex.

Gloves should also be pyrogen-free, as pyrogens can induce pyrexia and misdiagnosis in some patients. This fact is also well documented.

Powder-free, latex-free synthetic gloves should also be available for:

- wearers who are known to be type 1 latex allergic (and therefore prone to anaphylactic shock);
- patients who may be at higher risk of latex allergy (such as those with spina bifida, previous atopy, dermatitis, asthma or food allergies) or those who have undergone multiple surgical procedures.

These gloves should be of the same high quality as latex gloves, allowing comfort and sensitivity, and must be part of a total protocol within a surgical unit to eliminate risk to sensitised individuals.

Glove puncture is commonplace during surgery and occurs in over 50% of cases in some operative procedures. Studies show that between 50% and 92% of perforations pass undetected. Therefore, for many procedures (eg some orthopaedic, cardiac or gastrointestinal procedures) it would be prudent to double-glove using a green under-glove to ensure added protection. The use of two surgical gloves has been shown to maintain the barrier between the wearer and patient in four out of five cases in which the outer glove has been breached. Double gloving with a darker colour underglove will allow early identification of glove punctures. The size of the inner glove depends on the wearer but is often a half size larger to optimise sensitivity, dexterity and comfort. If the outer glove is punctured, fluid penetrates between the two gloves and a dark green patch alerts the wearer that a puncture has occurred and the outer glove can then be replaced.

In summary therefore, a surgeon should choose a glove that:

- is suitable for the surgical procedure;
- fits well and does not lose its shape or integrity;
- offers optimum sensitivity and durability;
- is powder-free;
- contains low levels of latex allergens and residual accelerators and is pyrogen free;
- is powder-free and synthetic for those with an allergy to natural rubber latex.

Powder-free, latex-free gloves should also be available for suitable emergency cases.

Acknowledgements

The Royal College of Surgeons of England *Surgical Skills for Students* development group

Rory McCloy

Bill Thomas

John Weston Underwood

Louise Goldring

Please note

While every effort has been made to ensure the accuracy of the information contained in this publication, no guarantee can be given that in its compilation all errors and omissions have been excluded. Readers wishing to use this information are recommended therefore to verify the facts for themselves when appropriate.

Photography by the RCS Photographic Studio

Design by Chatland Sayer, London

Typesetting by the RCS Publications Department

Illustrations by Oxford Designers and Illustrators Limited

Printed by Latimer Trend & Company, Plymouth